Diary of a
FAT
housewife

Shirley Cook

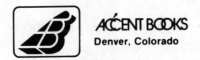

ACCENT BOOKS
Denver, Colorado

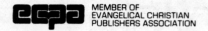 MEMBER OF
EVANGELICAL CHRISTIAN
PUBLISHERS ASSOCIATION

ACCENT BOOKS
12100 W. Sixth Avenue
P.O. Box 15337
Denver, Colorado 80215

Library of Congress Catalog Card Number: 77-71003

ISBN 0-916406-65-2

Daily Entries

Dedication

To Etta Hoffschneider
my Weight Watcher lecturer
and a lovely Christian

The End

W hat a way to start a book!
But won't you stop and take a look?
You've finally seen you're overweight,
But all those diets—you simply hate.

Well, good news! This isn't just another diet book; it's a *do-it* book; one that will inspire you to start, then stay with whichever diet you choose until you reach your goal. That's why THE END must come before the beginning.

THE END

of bad eating habits. In the past, we've eaten whatever, whenever and forever, knowing we would get fat. So we have to change our eating habits. We must learn good nutrition as well as proper quantities. I think the Weight Watchers' program meets these requirements. (I'm one of those who reached the goal, became a Lifetime member, then after a while, let old habits creep back in. And now I find that I have to start over again.) Maybe this has happened to you, and you feel like a failure, but you're not—you can be a winner!

Even if you're unable to attend Weight Watchers' meetings, you can follow the program in their cookbook found in most bookstores. Or if, for some reason, your doctor (be sure you see him before beginning any diet) believes you'd do better on a different plan, follow his instructions.

THE END

of living for self. This book may encourage and entertain you, but it can also be a source of eternal benefit if you have a personal relationship with Jesus Christ. Now wait, don't back off; give me a chance to explain.

You see, the Bible says that God loves you and has great plans for you. "For God so loved the world [you] that he gave his only begotten Son, that whosoever [you] believeth in him should not perish, but have everlasting life" (John 3:16). (Sounds good so far, doesn't it?)

Then we learn that man is sinful and separated from a holy God, so there's no way he can know and experience God's love and plan for his life. "For all have sinned and come short of the glory of God" (Romans 3:23). (We've missed the mark.)

But God has made a way to get us across this chasm (like a bridge over the Grand Canyon).

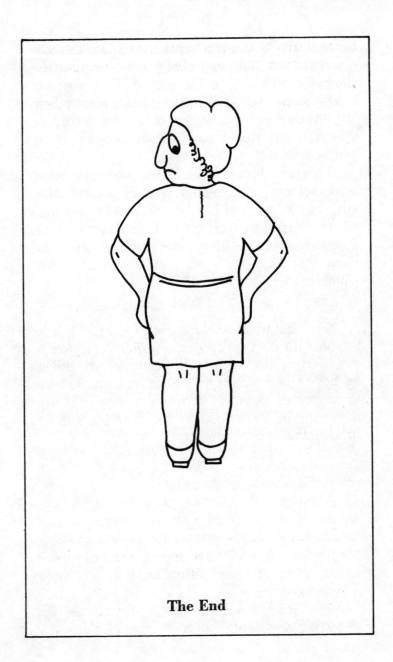

The End

He sent His Son, Jesus Christ, as the only provision for sin. Through Him, alone, because He alone was sinless, you can personally experience God's plan and love. "But God commendeth his love toward us, in that while we were yet sinners, Christ died for us" (Romans 5:8). (Can you believe it?)

To know Jesus Christ in this way, you must do something; receive Him (just as you would a gift) as Saviour and Lord by personal invitation. "But as many as received him, to them gave he power to become the sons of God, even to them that believe on his name" (John 1:12). (What a life!)

Now that we have considered THE END, let's get on with it. You may read a diary entry each day, every other day or once a week, depending on how much weight you have to lose. Be sure to memorize the daily scripture verses, taking advantage of *More Food for Thought*, because we need all the help we can get.

As *Tiny* Tim said in "The Christmas Carol," "God bless us, everyone!"

The Naked Truth

(Strength)

Dear Diary

"It can't be," I choked, ripping off my pink nylon nightie, and cautiously stepping on the "monster" once more. TWENTY pounds overweight. "Maybe it's my jewelry," I mumbled, as I removed my pierced earrings and small (it looks bigger in the light) diamond.

Those same horrible numbers still seemed to scream, "You're fat and getting fatter by the minute!"

It must be true, because I had to put one foot on the floor before the dial pointed to my ideal weight, and as it wasn't practical to get rid of my leg, I'd have to face it—another diet!

Well, I consider myself a professional dieter, although I've always received my pay in pounds rather than dollars. But which one should I try this time?

Grapefruit? Too sour. High protein?

Too much water. Ski team? Too boring. Low carbohydrate? Too much figuring. Vegetarian? Too green. Cottage cheese? Too white. I'd tried them all at least once, with little or no results. I couldn't stand them long enough to lose weight. If only someone would invent a diet that would allow you to eat all you want, and still lose a pound a day. "Oh, that would be—glory for me."

Last week I counted calories, but unfortunately, math was never my best subject, and I gained four pounds.

I know that to get the weight off and keep it off, I'll have to follow a sensible diet. So I'm getting out my favorite and starting on it today.

I'm already beginning to tremble, because as any compulsive eater knows, looking ahead to even a week of dieting brings on withdrawal pains, accompanied by stomach growls and twitching lips, and to contemplate dieting for more than a month might as well be eternity. That's my biggest problem. Can I stick to it? No matter how well-balanced and tasty a diet is, staying with it until I reach the goal is the real test.

I know how weak I am when it comes to food. I need strength outside myself. I need the Lord. He has shown Himself to be powerful in so many areas of my life. When I first trusted Him as Saviour over twenty years ago, He gave me strength

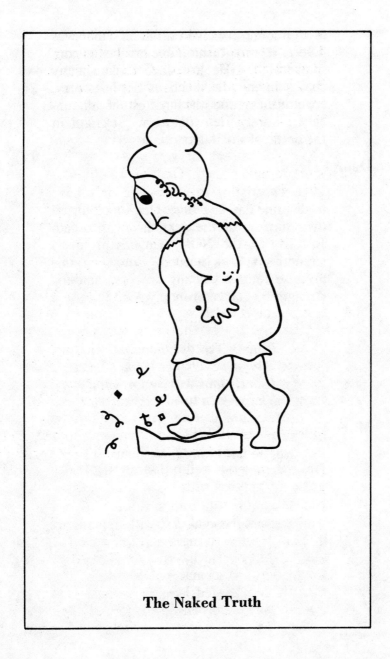

The Naked Truth

to overcome my cigarette habit (that was before it was fashionable to be a non-smoker), and He has since broken many chains in my life, such as doubt, worry, covetousness and the greatest of all, unbelief. Surely He will be my strength in the battle of the bulge too.

Dear Friend

Let's do this together—we only have to diet one day at a time. Don't look ahead to tomorrow or the next day with dread. Just live in the NOW. He has promised strength as it is needed. Count on this promise today, "As thy day, so shall thy strength be" (Deuteronomy 33:25).

Dear Lord

I thank You for the promise
That my every need You'll meet.
I surely look to You for help,
'Cause You know I love to eat!

More Food for Thought

"But be not thou far from me, O Lord: O my strength, haste thee to help me" (Psalm 22:19).

"I can do all things through Christ which strengtheneth me" (Philippians 4:13).

Mirror, Mirror,
on the Wall

(Appearance)

Dear Diary

"It's unfortunate that everyone can't see me just from the neck up," I said to the bathroom mirror. I looked around apprehensively, knowing that to get out of the bathroom, I would have to pass the full-length mirror attached to the door.

I usually managed to be rubbing my eyes or buttoning something as I left, or occasionally I backed up until I reached the door; but this morning, I decided to take a look. After all I'd stayed on the diet 100% yesterday. Maybe I looked good enough to cheat just a little today. Edging my way around the room and finally reaching my destination, I leaped in front of the mirror. Ta da! Gasp!

Was that fat lady standing there really me? Yes, there was the same face I'd seen just a few minutes before. But all of that substance attached to my neck, go-

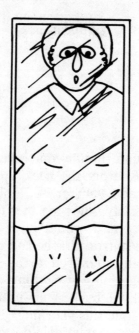

Mirror, Mirror, on the Wall

ing south? The only way I could see my whole body was in two installments.

Talk about an eye-opener! I thought of the scripture that says, "Beholding as in a glass, the glory of the Lord." I didn't see His glory reflected in my glass. I saw my own lack of discipline and moderation. Is this what others see too? Is my overweight a hindrance in reaching my friends for Christ?

That same verse goes on to say that we "are changed into the same image from glory to glory, even as by the Spirit of the Lord."

I believe that means that the more we behold Him through His Word, the more we'll be like Him. And all of this is accomplished by the Holy Spirit working in our lives.

Just as I should look in my mirror from time to time to get a true picture of myself, I should also look into the Bible for a true picture of Jesus. Then trusting Him and His power in my life, the Holy Spirit will make my character more like His.

Dear Friend

It's hard to see ourselves as others see us, but the mirror doesn't lie—unless it's in a funhouse. But looking deeply into God's Word will change us on the inside, and can't help but show through on the outside. What a promise today's verse is! "But we all, with open face beholding as in a glass, the glory of the Lord, are changed into the same image from glory to glory, even as by the Spirit of the Lord" (II Corinthians 3:18).

Dear Lord

*As I look within Your Word
And see Your Son revealed,
I bow in shame for my sin
In keeping Him concealed.*

More Food for Thought

"Therefore, if any man be in Christ, he is a new creature: old things are passed away; behold, all things are become new" (II Corinthians 5:17).

"And that ye put on the new man, which after God is created in righteousness and true holiness" (Ephesians 4:24).

What's
Eatin' You?

(Anger)

Dear Diary

Those girls! If they don't start picking up their clothes before they go to school, I'm gonna, I'm gonna . . . I'm gonna go get something to eat! And that husband of mine . . . why doesn't he understand me? I didn't mean to back into the electric garage door. How could I hear it going down with the baby crying at the top of her lungs? Boy, I feel like crying too. I feel like . . . like . . . eating. And why doesn't the choir director ever call on me to sing solos? Just because I can't hit a middle C! No one understands me.

I'm beginning to realize how I got into the habit of eating so much. I didn't know what else to do about my anger; after all, Christians shouldn't be angry, should they? I've always tried to swallow my anger— along with a big helping of something sweet. Keep up the smile—the pretense.

People think of me as that sweet (little?) thing who is always smiling. But it has hurt me to smile when underneath I was frowning. I've eaten to cover up, and have put on so much excess weight, I've probably shortened my life by several years.

But what can I do about it now? There will be times when my family makes me angry. And there will be instances when my friends and fellow Christians upset me. How can I handle it? Should I blow up, and tell everyone off? Should I stomp my feet and rage (primal scream) and let people know just what I think, regardless of how it may affect them?

I read a little article that said, "We often eat because of something that is eating us." And I believe that's been one of my problems. But the Bible teaches a more creative way to deal with anger than suppressing it, or expressing it. And that is confessing it.

Where does anger come from? I think it must be the response of a thwarted self-will. Now I'm not speaking of the duty of training children to be obedient. They must be disciplined, but believe it or not, it can be done without anger. I'm not talking about those disagreements between husband and wife that can be discussed calmly before coming to a solution. Nor am I thinking of a misunderstanding between friends that should be resolved

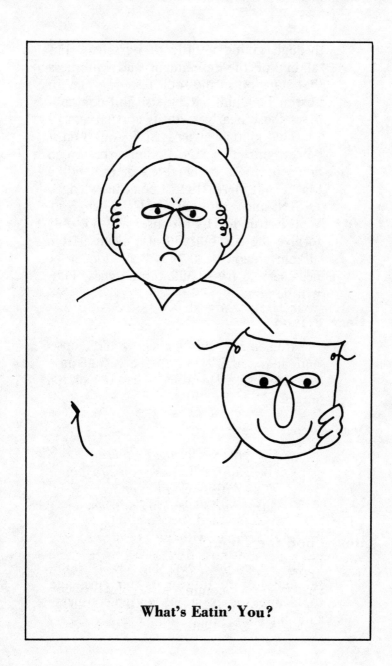

What's Eatin' You?

through giving a little of ourselves. I'm talking of the resentment and bitterness that stays on in the soul, festering like an unseen boil, until it bursts, and contaminates those nearby with its corruptness.

That kind of anger is SIN. And it must be recognized as SIN. It cannot be forced down by food, or laughter, or pretending that it isn't there. It must be acknowledged as SIN, and confessed as SIN. Then God, Who is true to His promise, will not only forgive the sin, but will also cleanse from all unrighteousness. It will no longer be necessary to try to hide those uglies. They will be gone.

Dear Friend

Remember this—when you're upset and angry, don't run to the refrigerator; run to Jesus. He alone can control our anger.

Dear Lord

Forgive me for the pretense
When I should have come to You
To confess my sin of anger
And find your promise true.

More Food for Thought

"If we confess our sins, he is faithful and just to forgive us our sins, and to cleanse us from all unrighteousness" (I John 1:9).

Watch Out!

(Decision)

Dear Diary

Obscene words from the corner of the
room startled me. "Go get something to
eat with a big glass of milk," they said.
"How about a big piece of chocolate cake,
or gooey apple pie? Maybe a hunk of
fudge or a thick sandwich?"

It was bad enough to hear those sug-
gestive words, but then pictures of rich
moist cake and yummy, crunchy potato
chips assailed my eyes.

Before I could turn off the TV, my
mouth began to water, my heart began
to pound, and I glanced furtively over my
shoulder. I knew I was alone because of
my sitting-up-late habit. (In the past, I
spent that time eating.) My puzzled husband, Les, had often said, "Honey, I don't
understand how you gain so much weight,
you hardly eat a thing." Ha. Little did he
know.

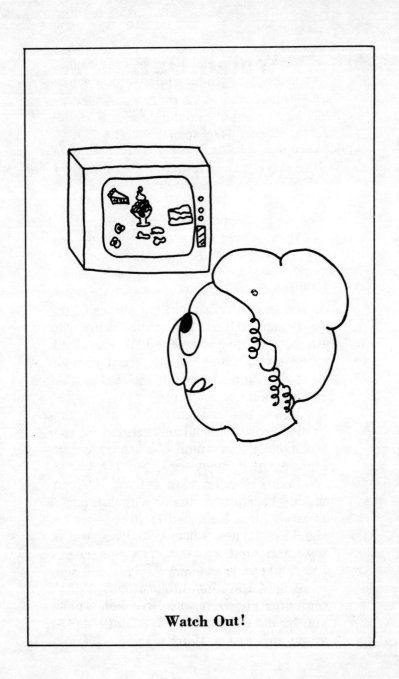

Watch Out!

Well, I was safe; no one was around, and a tiny little indulgence wouldn't matter. I heard the quiet rhythmic breathing of sleeping family coming from the bedrooms. Quietly tip-toeing to the "frig," I remembered one of the girls hadn't eaten all of her chocolate pudding at dinner. I could say if she asked about it, "Oh, it looked all dried out, so I got rid of it." That would be the truth.

As I opened the door, the light from inside revealed my fat hips, and I suddenly remembered I wasn't alone. God was watching. "The eyes of the Lord are upon the righteous . . ."

No, I couldn't do it. Not when I'd prayed that very morning that He would help me to stay on the diet. And He had —all day. Now, here I was, about to give in. But God . . . in His faithfulness, stopped me before I reached for that bowl.

To me, that small instant of time between conviction and obedience is like tottering on a high wire; but once your eyes are set on the goal, moving along in the right direction is not only easy, it's ecstasy!

And, oh joy, when I stepped on the scale this morning, it had moved down. I can almost detect a waistline.

Now I look forward to another day, committed to Him and His will, knowing that even when I'm alone and tempted to do the wrong thing, He is with me.

He is watching, not because He is an angry policeman-God, but because He is a loving Father-God. Isn't that great?

Dear Friend

God loves you with all His heart; so much that He can't keep His eyes off you. He really cares, not only about the things that seem important to others, but about the things that concern you. Trust Him today. He is watching; He hears. Let Him in on your problems. He can do something about them. He speaks for Himself, "The eyes of the Lord are upon the righteous, and his ears are open unto their cry" (Psalm 34:15).

Dear Lord

I thank You for the promise
That You're always watching me
And pray that I may give You
And others, something good to see.

More Food for Thought

"Doth not he see my ways, and count all my steps?" (Job 31:4).

"His head and his hairs were white like wool, as white as snow; and his eyes were as a flame of fire" (Revelation 1:14).

Dollars to Doughnuts

(Failure)

Dear Diary

Yesterday I goofed!

I was doing great until about 3 P.M., when I decided it would be fun to look in the store at some of the latest fashions and imagine the "new me" in some swingy mod outfit. I had to walk past the bakery to reach the department store, and had made up my mind, before leaving the car, that I would keep my eyes on my destination and not even sneak a tiny glance at the goodies in the window.

Walking with eyes straight ahead posed no problem, but I found it embarrassing to hold my nose in public, so was caught unaware by the aroma that floated out the door as a pleasingly plump patron passed through. The warm, sweet fragrance of fresh doughnuts drifted into my nostrils, causing my mouth to water and my stomach to growl simultaneously. Turning to snatch a quick look inside, I felt my body jerk an about face as my legs strode boldly into the store, dragging my weak will behind.

I only spent three minutes there—and five dollars! But the onion rolls would be perfect for our company dinner on Friday, and the children would love the cinnamon buns for breakfast. The pound cake would go into the freezer for an emergency and . . . after all, I deserved a doughnut for staying on my diet so well.

Unfortunately, when the doughnut was gone, all I had left was sugar on my chin, a sinking feeling in my heart and an extra lump on my hips.

Who did I think I was fooling anyway?

So I have to face myself again today. Do I really want to lose weight, or do I want to get fatter and fatter? Boy, some alternative.

Okay. I feel awful—guilty and weak-willed, but I can't bury my head in the refrigerator. I've got to get up and start again. Who said I'd never slip? I think I understand how the Apostle Paul felt when he wrote the seventh chapter of Romans. "Oh wretched man that I am! Who shall deliver me from the body of this death?"

Then came the glorious answer. "I thank God through Jesus Christ our Lord."

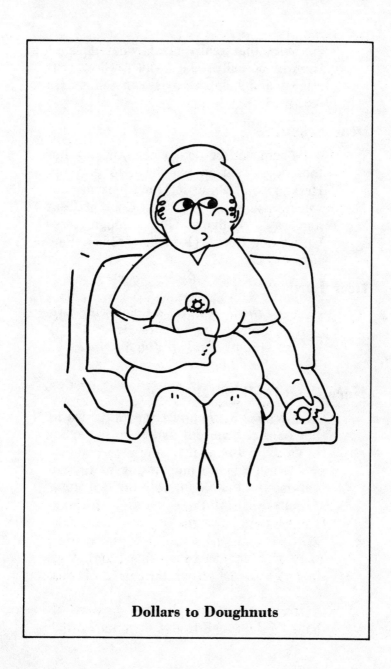

Dollars to Doughnuts

Does that really mean what it says? He will actually take away my low self-esteem and help me to see myself as He sees me?

Dear Friend

There will be days when you fail, but that doesn't mean you have to give up. He knows all about it. Don't look at your weakness and hate yourself. Look at Jesus and say, "I thank God through Jesus Christ our Lord" (Romans 7:25a). Fantastic!

Dear Lord

I thank and praise You for the love
You always have for me.
And as I look to You for grace
You'll be my victory.

More Food for Thought

"Who is he that overcometh the world, but he that believeth that Jesus is the Son of God" (I John 5:5).

"Restore unto me the joy of thy salvation; and uphold me with thy free spirit" (Psalm 51:12).

28

Weight for Me

(Misunderstanding)

Dear Diary

"Hey, kid, how about meeting me for lunch today? My treat."

"Sure," I answered, before she could change her mind. Bertha and I have had lots of fun together, mostly in all-you-can-eat places and ice cream parlors.

We always laughed behind the backs of those skinny people who picked at their food. Then I remembered the DIET.

"S'pose we could eat someplace different today? I think I'd better stay away from "The Trough."

"Oh, yeah, how come?"

"Well, guess what? I'm on a diet. And I've already lost enough weight that the clerk in the grocery store asked, "When did you have your baby?"

SILENCE—DEAD SILENCE—

"Why?" she blurted, as if I'd offended her. "I liked you as you were."

"Well—uh. . . "

"I guess we can't have fun anymore, then, if you're going to be on a diet."

"Of course we can," I assured her. "I still eat. Lots of good things like fruits and vegetables; anyway we don't have to be eating to have fun, do we?"

"No hot fudge sundaes?"

"No."

SILENCE. . .

"Oh, hey, I just noticed I've got a dentist's appointment today. We'll make it another time, okay?"

She hung up!

I couldn't believe it. Was our friendship only stuck together with hot fudge? I really like Bertha. She's always laughing and joking. But I guess down inside, she feels like me—kind of insecure about her size. I wondered if I should call her back and say that I'd go off my diet for a day. After all, she was one of my best friends. But how about Jesus? Could I turn my back on Him and what He wants of me just so others will accept me? No. He has helped me this far; I'll just have to go all the way.

Dear Friend

You may find that the business of losing weight is even harder than you thought it would be. It might mean the temporary loss of some of your friends. But let's remember, although there may

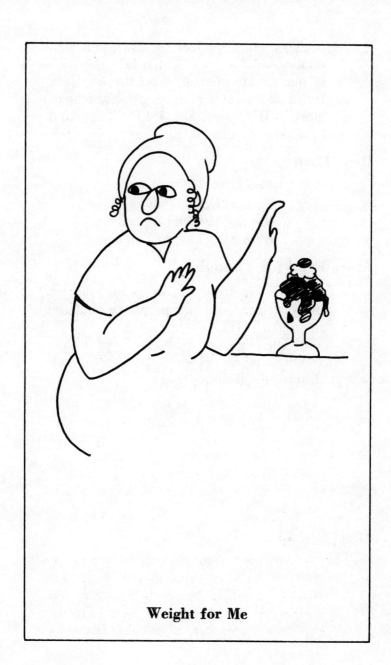

Weight for Me

be days when we feel let down and misunderstood, ". . . our light affliction, which is but for a moment, worketh for us a far more exceeding and eternal weight of glory" (II Corinthians 4:17). That kind of weight, we can take.

Dear Lord

You know how hard it is
To say "No" to those we love
But the blessings supersede
With our "Yes" to You above.

More Food for Thought

"We are troubled on every side, yet not distressed; we are perplexed, but not in despair" (II Corinthians 4:8).

"Then they cried unto the Lord in their trouble, and he delivered them out of their distresses" (Psalm 107:6).

In Due Season

(Perseverance)

Dear Diary

50% OFF!

The ad in the paper caught my eye. Hmm, swim suits. It had been a long time since I'd owned one, but maybe, just maybe, next season I'll be ready to make my debut.

Of course, I wouldn't be getting in the water, being a non-swimmer (I was glad to hear Ann Landers shares my problem). In fact, the water scares me so much, I wear a specially-designed shower cap with a built-in snorkle. Anyway, after weighing this morning, I felt so thin that I decided to take a look at those suits.

There was a good selection, but I really had to scrounge to find one with more than a half yard of material. I used to wear a size 12, and hoped to eventually get down to that size again, so I picked out a shocking pink, one-piece number, and slipped into the dressing room, avoiding the clerk with her eyes rolled up in her head.

"Ow . . . uh . . . grunt . . . puff . . . whew!" I tried to compose myself and wait until I could breathe again before turning to look in the mirror.

50% OFF—and more!

There was more of me out than in. My eyes began to sting and I suddenly felt nauseated. PHOOEY. I'd never be thin. I decided then and there to forget about the diet and go get something good to eat. It would be more fun to be fat and happy than half-fat and miserable.

"In due season we shall reap—if we faint not."

I looked around. Who said that?

Oh, yeah, I learned that verse once, but thought I'd forgotten it. And here the Lord was bringing it back to my memory. ". . . if we faint not."

Dear Friend

Just as it took months perhaps years to put on all that extra weight you're carrying around, it's going to take awhile to get rid of it. But you will—if you don't give up. Think about this verse when you feel like throwing in the scale, and you'll find not only a growing perseverance but also a shrinking body. "In due season we shall reap, if we faint not" (Galatians 6:9).

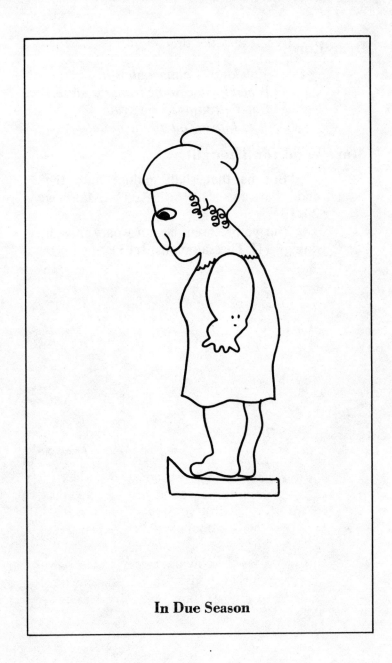

In Due Season

Dear Lord

You know I almost blew it
When I came home from the store,
But You stopped me again
And I love You all the more!

More Food for Thought

"But he that shall endure unto the end, the same shall be saved" (Matthew 24:13).

"But ye brethren, be not weary in well doing" (II Thessalonians 3:13).

Forbidden Fruit

(Temptations)

Dear Diary

My hands reached instinctively to my throat as I stepped back from the door, and braced myself against the wall. I certainly hadn't expected what I saw there —a big plate of steaming hot, sticky, pecan rolls, fresh from my neighbor's oven.

I tried to regain my composure, when I noticed Donna's concerned expression. "What's the matter, dear? I thought you and I could have some fresh rolls. Got some coffee on?"

"Oh—a—sure—come on in, Donna," I said, leading the way into an anything-but-neat kitchen. I was ready for a cup of coffee before tackling the syrup in the sink, the catfood in the corner and the toast under the table. But rolls? What could I say, so I wouldn't offend Donna?

"Oh, the rolls are beautiful, and look delicious. I know the family will love them;

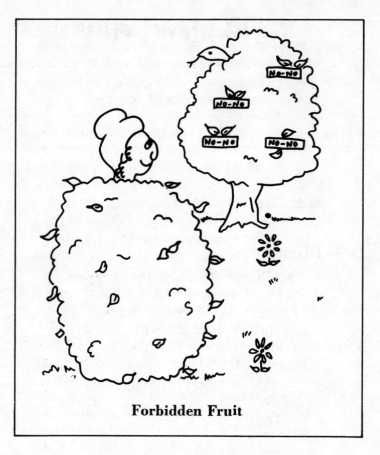

Forbidden Fruit

but you know I'm allergic to sweets." (I
break out in fat.)

"Oh, come on, I've seen you eat sweets
lots of times!"

"Well, to be honest, I'm trying to lose
weight, and I've got a long way to go."

"Then it won't hurt to eat them, just
this once. Come on, try them. How can it
really matter, that much?"

I looked yearningly at them. The longer I stared, the more sense her argument made. One or two rolls wouldn't make that much difference. I'd just be extra careful the rest of the day.

Funny. The whole scene struck a familiar chord. Oh, yes, the Garden of Eden.

Eve had everything a woman could want, except possibly a larger wardrobe. Her husband, an executive botanist-zoologist, loved her. She was healthy (probably had a great tan), ate fresh fruit and vegetables from her own garden, and above all, each evening, she had the pleasure of walking and talking with God. He had put her on a very special diet; He knew what would be bad for her, and she stuck to it pretty well. That is, until one day when this creepy character came along and in an oh-so-kind voice said, "God doesn't really mind if you eat that forbidden fruit. Anyway, how could it hurt?"

Eve looked and looked at it. It sure was tempting. In fact, it looked better than anything else in all the garden. "Adam would like it too," she thought. "Well, maybe, just this once. . . ."

I pulled my eyes away from the plate. "Donna, I know you like me, or you wouldn't have brought these rolls. I hope you like me well enough to let me refuse them this time. But I will have coffee with you, and you can tell me how good they are!"

We had a pleasant visit. She did understand, and I think that from now on, she will help me get down to my formerly fine figure.

Dear Friend

The temptation to give in to the allurements of the world is always a problem to the Christian; not only in the matter of diets, but in other things, such as our reactions to our families and our obedience to God in our everyday walk. And we don't have the power within our own natures to resist. But we do have God's promise in I John 4:4, "Ye are of God, little children, and have overcome them: because greater is he that is in you, than he that is in the world." We can resist the Tempter, as we look to the Saviour.

Dear Lord

Help me turn away
From the things I shouldn't crave
And to look up to Jesus
For He alone can save.

More Food for Thought

"There hath no temptation taken you but such as is common to man: but God is faithful, who will not suffer you to be tempted above that ye are able: but will with the temptation also make a way to escape, that ye may be able to bear it" (I Corinthians 10:13).

Hungover

(Depression)

Dear Diary

Yep, it's true. I have a hangover this morning (in more ways than one). My face looks like a creampuff, my arms feel like two giant sausages, my stomach is as bloated as a pregnant whale, and I can only move my feet about three centimeters per minute (have to get used to the new measuring system, you know). Shocking, huh? A nice middleclass Christian wife and mother waking up with a hangover. Oh, did I mention . . . it wasn't alcohol that did this to me? It was food.

Yes, it's a fact. I went on a binge yesterday, an eating binge. It started with a not-too-serious disagreement at the breakfast table. By the time everyone had left for work and school, I felt depressed. Needless to say, I didn't get MY way in the argument. But I didn't want to pray about my reactions—I was right. So to nurture my wounded pride, I decided to finish up a piece of leftover toast, adding a little honey, of course. "Hmm, that tasted pretty good. I think I'll have another, and another." Before I realized it, I had eaten FOUR slices of toast, decorated with such colorful toppings as peanut butter and jam, honey and bananas and finally maple syrup (which I hate). Something had "clicked" in my brain, and my whole body went out of control. The more I ate, the more depressed I became, and the more I ate. It didn't end at breakfast. I ate all day—everything I had stayed away from so faithfully. Candy bars, ice cream, potato chips, ad infinitum.

By bedtime, I felt so sick physically and spiritually that I couldn't even look up to my heavenly Father and ask His forgiveness.

Where did it all begin? Why did I do it?

My guard had been down when I went to the breakfast table yesterday morning. I was tired when I got up, because I foolishly stayed up for the late show (I used to do that so I could eat). And when I started to hassle my son about the way he wears his hair, the rest of the family came to his defense. Would you believe it? I probably wouldn't have brought it up if I'd taken that tiny instant to seek God's will, but no, I just had to speak my mind. It wasn't a serious matter, but I made it serious, because I wasn't willing to depend upon the guidance of the Holy Spirit.

I think I've learned something from this experience; disobedience to God brings on depression, and depression, to an obese personality, brings on a food binge.

Well, it's a new day, and I'm still tired. But am I tired enough? I'm tired of carrying around all this extra weight. I'm tired of feeling like a failure; tired of making

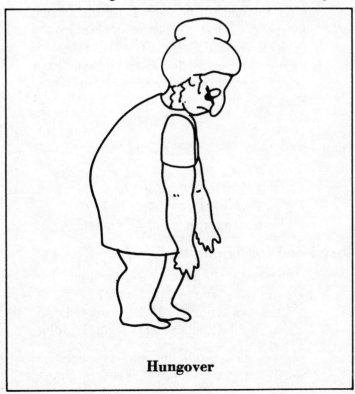

Hungover

excuses; tired of being in a rut; tired of fooling myself. I'm tired of being self-centered, and tired of trying instead of trusting. But am I really tired enough to let go, and let God?

Dear Friend

I hope you don't fall into this unnerving situation that I've just been through; but if you do, remember, don't reach for food when you feel depressed. Drop to your knees and confess your anxiety to God. He will lift you up. It is your choice to react to the problems of life in the flesh, or in the Spirit. Romans 8:8 says, "They that are in the flesh cannot please God." And I know you want to please Him, too.

Dear Lord

Thank You for this new day
That I may live for Thee.
Today I'll trust alone in YOU
Instead of depending on ME.

More Food for Thought

"Casting all your care upon him: for he careth for you" (I Peter 5:7).

"Let not your heart be troubled: ye believe in God, believe also in me" (John 14:1).

Under New Management

(Commitment)

Dear Diary

Whew! It's good to sit back and look at a job well done. Whoops—there's a piece of fuzz under the table! Well . . . almost done.

We're having friends over for dinner tonight, which is always an excuse (I shouldn't need one) to clean house extra good. It's not that I'm trying to make false impressions, it's just that I like for my friends to feel comfortable and welcome in our home, and those few extra swipes with the dust cloth, and fresh flowers on the tables will give them the feeling that I care, not only about my home, but also about them.

Sure hope they don't look in the hall closet. It's so full of everything from Monopoly minus money to Mother's mending mess, that we have nicknamed it the "City Dump." Who knows—umbrellas without

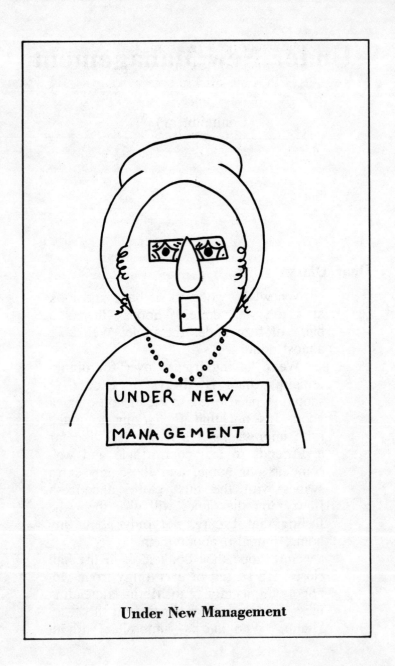

Under New Management

handles may be a fad someday. I suppose most people have certain "closets" in their homes that are off limits to casual friends, but open to close ones.

I wonder if I consider the Lord a close enough friend to give Him access to every part of my life? The Bible says, "Know ye not that ye are the temple of God, and that the Spirit of God dwelleth in you?" (I Corinthians 3:16).

When I trusted in Jesus as Saviour, the Holy Spirit moved in, and hung up the sign "Under New Management." I am His temple. Is it a place where He feels comfortable and welcome, or have I neglected it, and let it get run down, or overcrowded? Are there still hidden closets where He hasn't been given access? Like . . . my appetite? I think I'd better do some housecleaning in my temple so the Lord will know He is not only a welcome guest, but the permanent owner and resident.

Dear Friend

I don't know if it's good or bad to have so many articles on the market about overweight and why people are fat. We used to get away with the argument of heredity or metabolism. Now the psychologists have broadcast it to the world that we're fat because we have hang-ups.

I suppose one of the quickest ways to really get the temple in shape is to admit our weaknesses to ourselves (without self-hate) and turn them over to the Lord, Who alone knows us inside and out. He can conquer all our frustrations whether they began in childhood or whether they're new. Let's commit our whole being to Him —our bodies, which are His temple, our eyes, which are the window of our souls, and our mouths, which not only eat too much, but often say the wrong things. You and I are His; He bought us with His own blood.

"Set a watch, O Lord before my mouth; keep the door of my lips" (Psalm 141:3).

Dear Lord

I want to be Your temple
A place where You abide.
I give you now, free access
With nothing more to hide.

More Food for Thought

"What? know ye not that your body is the temple of the Holy Ghost which is in you, which ye have of God, and ye are not your own?

"For ye are bought with a price: therefore glorify God in your body, and in your spirit, which are God's" (I Corinthians 6:19-20).

A Real Winner

(Goals)

Dear Diary

It's exciting enough just to watch your number one son run on the track team, but it's really something else when he comes in number one in the race too.

"How does a person get to be a winner?" I asked him at dinner last night.

"Well, Mom, you've got to keep your eyes on the goal, and not look around at the other guys. When I'm running," he went on, "it's like I'm a different person. My whole concentration is on the goal. That's all I see in my mind's eye; even when the goal is actually out of sight, it's there in my imagination, and I'm there crossing it first."

Wow! I can see that if I want to succeed in this contest of thin versus fat, I'm going to have to keep my mind on the goal.

And what was that he said about

imagination? He pictured himself as winning. I came across the same thought in Tim LaHaye's book, *How to Win over Depression.* He said that if you get a mental picture of yourself as thin, your subconscious mind will lead you in that direction. I hate to admit that I've thought of myself as a weak-willed character when it comes to dieting, and therefore, I've been a weak-willed character. But by God's grace, I'm going to project a successful image of Diet No. 120.

My goal: To be thin. To be in control of my eating habits. To be God's person. I know it will be hard to keep my eyes on that goal. I always like to look around and see what others are doing, and in my family of "skinnies," they're usually eating.

And have you noticed that a runner can only take one step at a time? So it is with eating. It's one meal at a time; one day at a time. You have to keep your eyes on the goal, and run one step at a time.

Dear Friend

Have you set goals for your life? It's important if you expect to make any progress. So take a few minutes right now and set the final goal you want to reach on your weight loss program. Then set a realistic goal for each week (Oh, come on now, you know you can't lose ten pounds

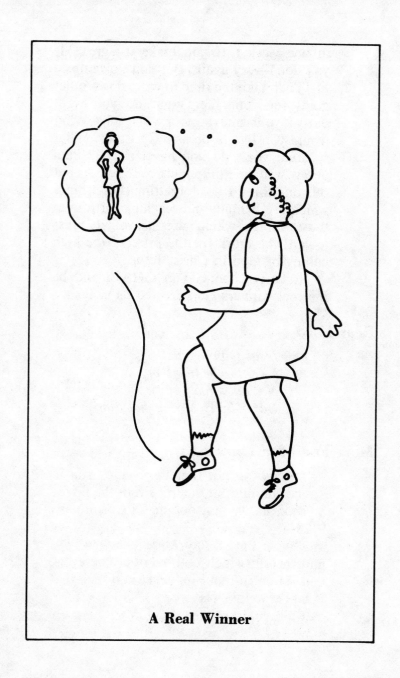

A Real Winner

in one week.) If you make it—great. If you don't—try again. But don't give up.

Then take the time to write down other goals for your life. What do you want out of your marriage or your job? What would you like to be as a Christian? What spiritual goals do you have, if any? Paul put it well in Philippians 3:13, ". . . but this one thing I do, forgetting those things which are behind, and reaching forth unto those things which are before, I press toward the mark for the prize of the high calling of God in Christ Jesus."

Let's put the GO in GOAL, and be the real winners God created us to be.

Dear Lord

Jesus is my goal
I want to be like Him.
Not only in my spirit,
But in body, strong and trim.

More Food for Thought

"Know ye not that they which run in a race run all, but one receiveth the prize? So run, that ye may obtain" (I Corinthians 9:24).

". . . Let us lay aside every weight, and the sin which doth so easily beset us, and let us run with patience the race that is set before us" (Hebrews 12:1).

An Impatient Patient

(Patience)

Dear Diary

Oooh, my head aches, my stomach cramps and my back is as stiff as raw spaghetti. I have the flu. I don't get sick very often, so I'll try to make the best of it. Let's see—if I just stay in bed, I can have people wait on me, and I won't have to do any of the work. Ooooh, I feel too lousy to enjoy my leisure. I even have a temperature.

That's rare for me, I'm usually subnormal (my temperature, that is). It was 100 degrees this morning, and dropped to 99.6 around noon, and now it's up to 102. I wonder what it will be an hour from now. I'll let you in on a secret I learned about myself—when I'm sick, I'm not only a compulsive weigher, but I'm also a compulsive temperature-taker.

I managed to get myself on the scale this morning right after taking my temp, then again a few minutes ago. It seems that I've lost a lot of weight. Ooooh, my head hurts. It's hard to remember details, but I think I weighed 102, and my temperature was over 140. Yes, that must be right. Wow, 102—I'm really going to look good when I get out of this sick bed. I guess it's worth it after all.

"Hey, somebody, will you bring me another dish of ice cream?"

Dear Friend

Well, I've recovered from the flu, and although it's wonderful to feel well again, I found, to my dismay, that I'd only lost ONE pound through all my suffering, which must prove something. I have to be more than a sickly patient to get rid of this weight, I have to be sick enough of my old ways to patiently learn new ways.

Remember the old saying about Rome not being built in a day? Well, me neither.

You and I must learn patience, and it doesn't come easily. But as we daily look to the God of all patience for strength to stay on our diets, we'll find, in time, that we have not only learned new eating habits, but that we also have slim new figures that are honoring to the God we serve.

So hang in there! There will be setbacks in our diets from time to time, just as there are in other realms of our lives, but it's through tribulation that we learn patience.

" . . . Be not slothful, but followers of them who through faith and patience inherit the promises" (Hebrews 6:12).

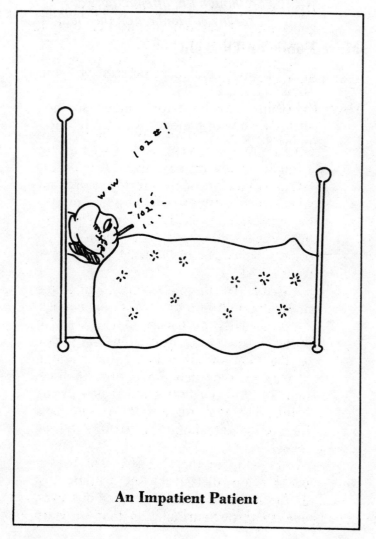

An Impatient Patient

Dear Lord

Patience is a virtue
Usually learned through trial.
So though I'm often hungry
I see lower numbers on the dial.

More Food for Thought

"In your patience possess ye your souls" (Luke 21:19).

"But if we hope for that we see not, then do we with patience wait for it" (Romans 8:25).

Signs and Wonders

(Fear)

Dear Diary

I wondered what that funny bump was on the side of my foot. I couldn't examine it as well as I wished while sitting in church; but continued to glance down as I half-heartedly listened to the closing remarks of the pastor. With the final "Amen," I casually reached down to touch the strange protrusion, and was surprised to find its twin poking out of my other foot. I drew back my hand in revulsion. What could it be?

I tried to hide my concern behind smiles and vigorous hand-shaking as we left the church; but underneath I felt a dread and fear of the unknown casting a shadow upon my future.

Not wanting to alarm the children, I waited until we were home to show my husband the "bumps."

"Darling," I said, unable to restrain

the quiver in my voice, "something is wrong with my feet, and I wonder if you have any idea what it could be the sign of." I braced myself and held up my "deformed" foot. He snickered, then broke into a fit of laughter. What was wrong with him? How could he be so insensitive? I may have been bitten by a rare spider, or have the beginnings of some dread disease.

"Honey," he said, patting me fondly, "those bumps are signs and wonders all right—they're your ankle bones—a sign that you're getting thin!"

Ankle bones? I wondered if they stuck out like that on other people. I'd never really given it much thought.

"Are you kidding? Let me see yours," I demanded. He pushed down his socks and sure enough, there they were, identical bumps to mine.

"Ankle bones!" I joined in the laughter as the children came in one by one to see what was so funny. And to think, I was afraid.

Well, to be perfectly honest, I am a little apprehensive of becoming thin. I don't really know why. I just have so many questions, like . . . will the change in my appearance bring about other changes in my life that I won't know how to cope with? Will people still regard me as the same person they've always known? Will I be more susceptible to hurts when I'm

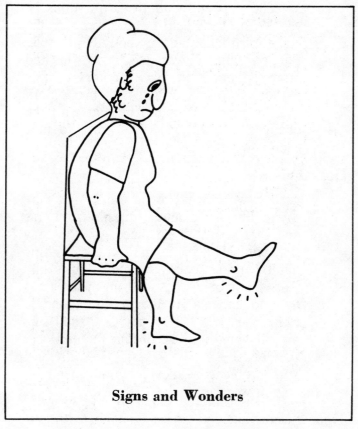

Signs and Wonders

no longer shrouded in a cloak of flesh?
I could hardly believe it. I *was* afraid—of
thinness. I would no longer be able to hide
my feelings under the expected joviality
of a fat person. I would have to face up
to my own fears and longings. How could
I accept my new position in society? People
would have to take me more seriously
than before. Could I adjust to these
changes in my life?

The answer to all these questions is, yes. With God's help I could, because the Holy Spirit had made my body His temple. Fat or thin, I was His, and He had promised never to leave or forsake me. My desire to lose weight is to bring glory to Him, and I'm confident that with the changes, He will give His grace to face each new situation.

Dear Friend

Are you afraid to be thin? That may sound like a ridiculous question, but it's one that needs to be faced, or you may find yourself back in the same old eating habits, trying to cover up the hurts and fears with extra flesh. Bring your fears to God and claim His promise found in Philippians 4:19, "But my God shall supply all your need according to his riches in glory by Christ Jesus." He will meet your problems as they come, not before—so quit worrying.

Dear Lord

I know I shouldn't be afraid
It really is a sin,
So I'll trust you now and then
Whether thick or thin.

More Food for Thought

"There is no fear in love; but perfect love casteth out fear: because fear hath torment. He that feareth is not made perfect in love" (I John 4:18).

Persistent Primate

(Habits)

Dear Diary

After slicing one inch from each end of the ham, I put it in the pan and popped it into the oven. "Mom," Christy said, watching my every movement, "why do you always cut off the ends of the ham?"

"Oh, I don't know, honey, it's just a habit. Your grandmother always did, so I thought I should too. I think I'll call her and find out the reason."

I hung up the phone and shrugged my shoulders. "She doesn't know either. She said her mother always did it. She's calling Great Grandma to ask her."

A few minutes later, the answer came. I felt my face redden as my mother laughed. "She said she cut off the ends of the ham—because her pan was too small!"

I had habitually prepared ham that way, ignorant of the reason, just as I habit-

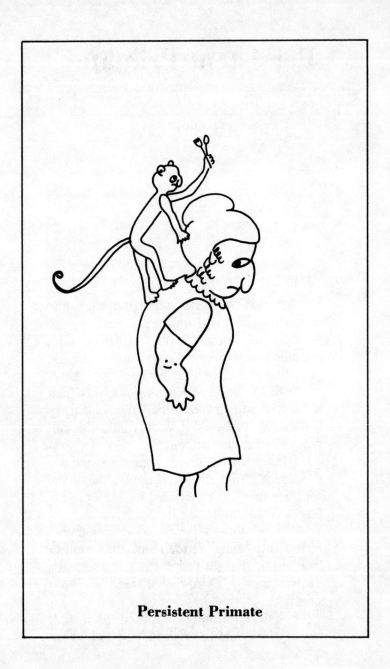

Persistent Primate

ually overate, not knowing why. I'm sure it will be easy to break the ham habit, but breaking the obesity habit seems almost impossible. It has become so strong from use that it borders on addiction.

Oswald Chambers says a habit dominates because it was willingly yielded to in the first place; and only by willingly yielding to Jesus Christ can the bondage of a bad habit be broken.

If I want to be permanently delivered from an overactive fork (not just till I reach my ideal weight), then there must be a deeper work done in my life, and Jesus Christ wants to do it.

Dear Friend

Are you having trouble getting that monkey off your back? You think you've gotten rid of him for awhile, then he jumps right on again. Humanly speaking, it's harder for us fatties to break the habit of overeating than for an alcoholic to break his habit. He gives up alcohol completely, while we must still eat three times a day. Even St. Augustine said, "Total abstinence is easier than perfect moderation." (I wonder if he shared our problem?)

But that just gives us a greater reason to yield everything, yes, even our appetites, to God. He alone can take that bad habit of overeating and keep it caged where it can no longer control us.

"The Lord shall deliver me from every evil work [habit] and will preserve me unto his heavenly kingdom" (II Timothy 4: 18a).

Dear Lord

For victory over a habit
There really is no lack,
For You are strong enough
To get it off my back!

More Food for Thought

". . . My grace is sufficient for thee: for my strength is made perfect in weakness" (II Corinthians 12:9a).

"Though he fall, he shall not be utterly cast down: for the Lord upholdeth him with his hand" (Psalm 37:24).

Sacrifice of Praise

(Praise)

Dear Diary

This dieting business really drags some days, and my very perceptive family sensed that I needed encouragement yesterday. This is what I got:

"Honey," Les said, putting his arm around me (well, not all the way around), "I can sure tell that you're losing weight."

"Oh, really?" I put my hands on my hips, wondering how he would compliment me.

"Sure, you know I used to have to hold on to the edge of the bed to keep from rolling toward the center—and I don't anymore." He smiled, pleased with his words of encouragement and praise.

Kathy was next with, "Oh, Mom, you don't look nearly as gigantic from the back anymore." A compliment? I think so.

Then my son decided he would praise me as I was groping my way toward the kitchen to fix breakfast (hair still in rollers

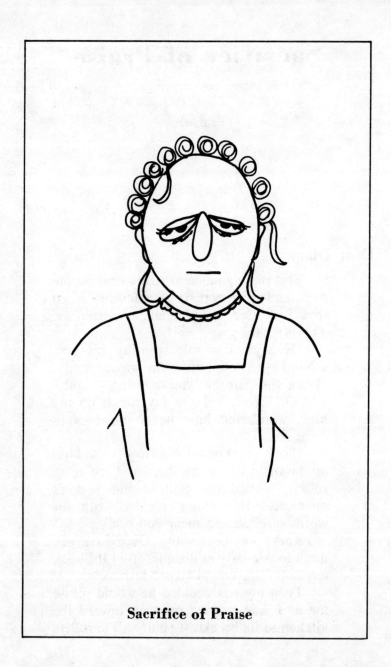

Sacrifice of Praise

and no make-up). "Mom, you sure do look better than you used to!"

This was what I call the sacrifice of praise. They saw that I was a little discouraged and tried to help. And I appreciate it. I know it came from their hearts. My diet didn't seem so hard after those words. At least my loved ones are aware that I'm working at it, and their encouragement is essential.

I love praise as much as the next person, and I don't even deserve it. But did you know God loves praise too? And He has it coming. It isn't always easy, on our part, to praise Him, especially when things aren't going the way we think they should; but love will find a way.

My family *hopes* that I'll keep my promise to stick with my diet, so they give praise to keep me going. But we *know* that God is going to do what He has promised, and we can praise Him with confidence.

Thank and praise Him for your weaknesses, because through them you can know His strength. Praise Him for your heartaches, for they can lead you to the Comforter. Praise Him for your fears; perfect love casts out fear. Praise Him for your troubles; it's an opportunity to grow in patience. We can praise Him for anything and everything, for He is the Author of Life and is workng all things together for our good. Praise the Lord!

Dear Friend

Take this occasion to offer the sacrifice of praise to the Lord. It not only pleases and honors Him, but you will find His power being released in your life as you do. You can't help but be happy when you are in the center of God's will; and those who praise Him, are.

I Thessalonians 5:18 says, "In everything give thanks [praise]: for this is the will of God in Christ Jesus concerning you."

Praise the Lord!

Dear Lord

You've made a promise
To guide me all my days,
And though it's sometimes difficult
I'll always give You praise.

More Food for Thought

"Rejoice in the Lord alway: and again I say, Rejoice" (Philippians 4:4).

"Let my mouth be filled with thy praise and with thy honor all the day" (Psalm 71:8).

Instant Everything

(Endurance)

Dear Diary

"What's for dinner tonight, honey?"
Les asked, poking his head into the kitchen
and wrinkling up his nose. "I don't see
anything cooking, and I don't smell anything either." He glanced at his watch.
"It's ten till six, isn't it?"

"Don't worry," I said over my
shoulder, "I'll have dinner ready in just
a few minutes. I had to listen to the 'News
Capsule' first."

I looked in the cupboard. Instant
macaroni and cheese, instant biscuits, instant coffee. "Good," I whispered, reaching for the freezer door. Instant gourmet-
style vegetables, instant onion rings, and
for desert, instant cherries jubilee. I shook,
dumped and placed each item in its proper
pan (some came with instant pans), and
while they boiled, baked and soaked, I
read my condensed version of "War and

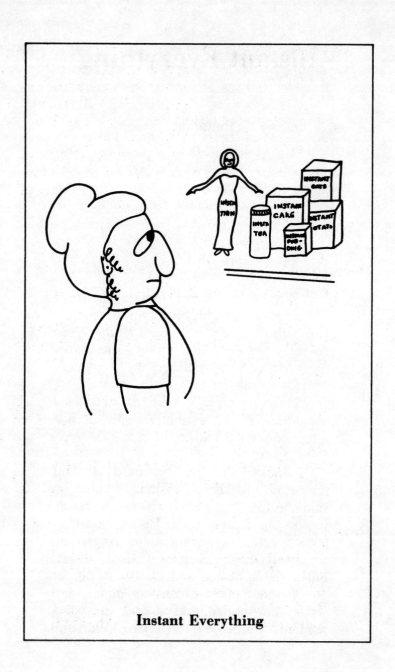

Instant Everything

Peace." Amazing that it could be squeezed into two chapters.

The family sat down and instantly devoured whatever it was on their plates, and disappeared just as instantly into various rooms, corners and cubby holes.

I sat alone at the table thinking about how quickly we move through life, hardly stopping to notice the things that were not developed instantly. How about mountains, oceans, flowers, vegetable gardens, good marriages and children with honorable characters? All these things take time to grow, and because of their long nurturing process, we hold them even more valuable.

I've been impatient about losing weight, too. I often become discouraged that it isn't faster. I could go on an instant diet and lose quickly, but I'd probably gain it back just as quickly—or I'd be too weak to know I was slim. Good things take time; yes, I'll have to develop some patience along the way. I didn't gain all this extra weight overnight, so I'd better give it time to come off too.

Dear Friend

In this age of instant food, instant cash, instant lawns and instant credit, try to remember that God isn't in a hurry. To Him one day is as a thousand years, and a thousand years is as one day; so as

His children, we too must learn patience, not only with others, but also with ourselves and our diets.

"They that wait upon the LORD shall renew their strength; they shall mount up with wings as eagles; they shall run, and not be weary; and they shall walk, and not faint" (Isaiah 40:31).

I wonder if there's a condensed version of the Bible?

Dear Lord

I hurry, hurry, hurry
Through each and every day.
So help me to slow down a bit
And LIVE along the way.

More Food for Thought

"I waited patiently for the LORD; and he inclined unto me and heard my cry" (Psalm 40:1).

"I must work the works of him that sent me, while it is day: the night cometh, when no man can work" (John 9:4).

Remember Lot's Wife

(Backsliding)

Dear Diary

TEN pounds of ugly, life destroying fat are gone. I've reached a midway point in my diet, and can hardly wait until that day when I'll be at goal.

Les has been such an attentive husband lately; he even took me to lunch to celebrate my success, and I thoroughly enjoyed it—and him. I went the salad and coffee route while he downed a cheeseburger, french fries and milk shake. It's amazing how he, a true skinny, can eat anything he wants and never gain a pound. Amazing? Disgusting is more like it.

I still have that old longing for something rich and gooey, and couldn't help overhear the lady in the booth behind me drool, "Isn't this the best hot fudge sundae you've ever eaten?" Hot fudge sundae. From then on, I could think of nothing else, even though Les was animatedly telling me of vacation plans.

Unable to control my curiosity any longer, I turned and looked over my shoulder. Oh, it did look good; thick, dark chocolate draped over white ice cream. I could almost taste the fluffy peaks of whipped topping that crowned the masterpiece. Maybe, since I'd already lost ten pounds, it would be all right to indulge in a "Fatty's Delight"!

Then I remembered Lot's wife.

Many years ago, a man named Lot took his wife and family to live in the beautiful, fertile valley of Sodom. How happy she must have been to be a citizen of Sodom after traveling around in the desert and living in drafty tents for several years. She probably joined right in with high society because the Bible says that Lot became a great leader in the community (and behind every great man, there's a great woman).

Her life was easy now—she had all the material possessions she'd gone without for so long. But Sodom was a wicked city, and God planned to destroy it.

He sent angels to lead Lot and his family to a safe place and to admonish them not to look back on Sodom, or yearn for those old worldly pleasures any longer.

Lot obeyed God, and set his eyes on the new land God had prepared for him; but his wife hated to give up the life she had come to love, and turned to take one last, longing look.

Oh, dread—she became a pillar of salt!

Surely a lesson can be learned from Lot's wife. I must look ahead to the new things the Lord has for me, and not look back with longing on my old habits of over-eating and self-indulgence.

If I do, I won't become a pillar of salt, but I will become a tub of lard.

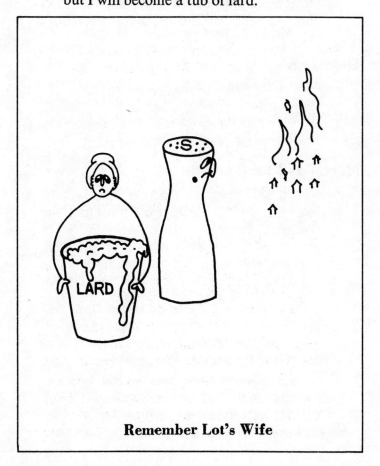

Remember Lot's Wife

Dear Friend

God gives us so many practical examples of living in the Bible. But the only way we can know them is to read His Word and determine, by His grace, to obey what we learn.

In this matter of looking back, Jesus even reminded those who followed Him to be careful about returning to their former behavior and to "Remember Lot's wife" (Luke 17:32).

Dear Lord

A pillar of the community
Was Lot's dear wife.
But I'd rather look ahead
And avoid that kind of strife.

More Food for Thought

"Look unto me, and be ye saved, all the ends of the earth: for I am God, and there is none else" (Isaiah 45:22).

"And Jesus said unto him, no man, having put his hand to the plough and looking back, is fit for the kingdom of God" (Luke 9:62).

First Things First

(Priorities)

Dear Diary

"What should I do first? I know I ought to have my quiet time with God; and the longer I leave the breakfast dishes, the stickier they'll become. The beds are unmade—the laundry is spilling out of the hamper, and I have some juicy news (okay, gossip) I'm dying to tell Brenda."

That was how my morning started. I decided to call Brenda first. Hmmph, I can't understand her attitude. She stuck up for Edith. Oh, well, see if I ever tell her anything again.

That was only the beginning of a day to be forgotten. While I was still on the phone, my mother-in-law dropped in, for "just a few minutes." Of course, she didn't look too impressed by the dishes piled in the sink, bread crumbs scattered across the table, and, "Oh, isn't that Becky's shoe?" under the couch. Then to complete

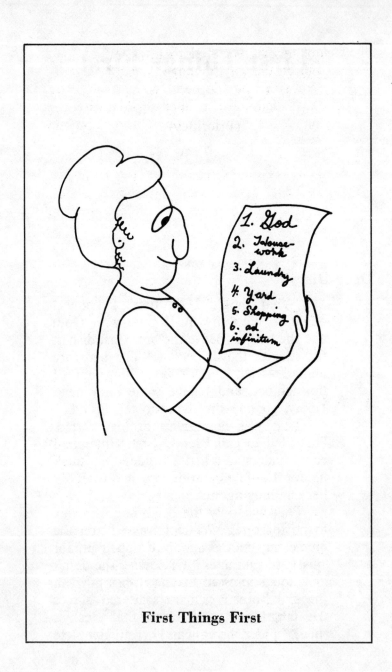

First Things First

my misery, she had to powder her nose, and on the way, managed to observe three rooms of unmade beds, with a variety of skirts and blouses intermingled with the blankets because, "I don't have anything to wear, Mom!"

I finally tackled the Monday Morning Mess and had things in good order by the time the gang swooped in after school, starving and ready to change clothes again!

P.S.   There never was a "Quiet Time."

My whole day was second-rate because I didn't put first things first. The Bible says that in all things Christ should have the preeminence (Colossians 1:18). And not giving Him prime time, I ended up not giving Him any time.

Dear Friend

It can be dangerous to leave Christ out of your day, for many reasons. But for the dieter, it's double danger. There are not only frustrations to deal with, but you may fall back on your old fluster-buster, food.

The Lord Jesus Christ didn't have this problem. He always had His priorities straight. Remember when He was in the wilderness for forty days and nights? That could have been a frustrating experience. He was hungry. He was lonely. He was tired. Then along came the Frustrator, himself, and told Jesus to look down on the ground. "See those stones?" he asked. The Lord could make them into bread if He wanted to. But He was already fortified with an awareness of His Father's presense, and bread, although it is not sinful in itself, was not what He needed. His food was to do the will of God, and that would never include obeying Satan, in any way.

Beginning now, let's start our days right—with God. The Creator of the Universe certainly deserves first place in our lives. As we live each day, conscious of His indwelling presence, we will find the words of Jesus true, "Man shall not live by bread alone, but by every word of God" (Luke 4:4).

Dear Lord

It's sometimes hard to seek You
At the outset of my day,
But life goes much smoother
If I first read the Bible and pray.

More Food for Thought

"If ye then be risen with Christ, seek those things which are above, where Christ sitteth on the right hand of God" (Colossians 3:1).

"I love them that love me; and those that seek me early shall find me" (Proverbs 8:17).

Three Cheers for Life

(Enthusiasm)

Dear Diary

If you had seen me yesterday, you would have seen a happier face on an iodine bottle. I was about ready to give up on my diet, drop my Sunday School class and burn my cookbook. I guess you could say I was down. That was when Karen called and asked me to come over for a cup of coffee. Those few minutes with her completely changed my outlook; she was so enthusiastic about life that it just splashed over on me, and today I feel like cheering!

She made me see how exciting it is to be a Christian. I saw by her home that she was even excited about housework. (I get excited about it too—but in a negative way.) Everything she touched seemed to have a glow. What made the difference?

ENTHUSIASM. She admitted that some days when she wakes up, she thinks,

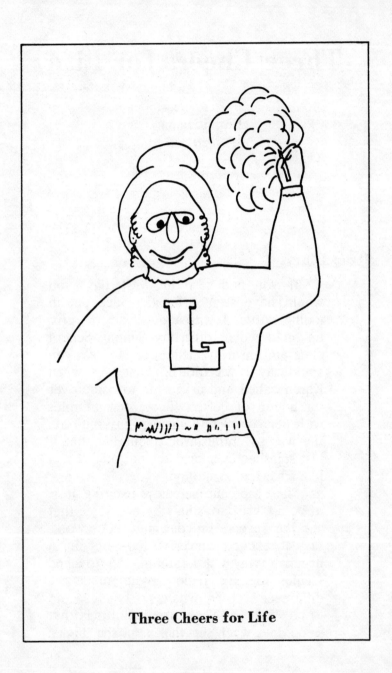

Three Cheers for Life

"Oh, no, not another day." But before she puts her feet on the floor, she prays, "Thank you, God, for another day!" She often has to force herself to be enthusiastic, but before long, she not only feels it, she is enthusiastic. And the secret lies within.

Our word enthusiasm comes from the Greek word, *entheos,* which means, "the god within." (I'm not a Greek student, just a voracious reader.) For the Christian, it is the *God* within. And what could make a person more enthusiastic about living than knowing and counting upon the actual presence of God within?

I want to be inspired in my life, and I want to inspire others, too. And I realize that not only is enthusiasm infectious—so is the lack of it. So watch out world—here I come. Boy, even that diet looks exciting to me; I know I'm going to reach my goal, and enjoy doing it!

Dear Friend

Why go about your work, your diet and your life half-heartedly? It makes it so hard. Get enthusiastic. Let the Holy Spirit put the sparkle in your days. The Bible says, "And whatsoever ye do, do it heartily, as to the Lord, and not unto men" (Colossians 3:23).

Don't just do whatever you're doing to please yourself or others, but do it for the Lord. And get that strain off your face. Smile. Do it HEARTILY. You'll be surprised how others' lives will be affected as you live this way. And God's Name will be glorified.

Dear Lord

Hurray! for the Holy Spirit
Who has come to live within.
Hurray! for my diet
Hurray! I'm getting thin!

More Food for Thought

"Finally, my brethren, be strong in the Lord, and in the power of his might" (Ephesians 6:10).

"And God is able to make all grace abound toward you; that ye, always having all sufficiency in all things, may abound to every good work" (II Corinthians 9:8).

Mind Over Platter

(Moderation)

Dear Diary

I almost didn't make it. Baked potatoes, oozing with sour cream; steak, smothered in mushroom sauce; hot rolls, all you could eat. And to top it off, French pastries.

You think this was a dream, maybe? I wish it were. In a dream, I could eat it all and not gain an ounce.

Mr. and Mrs. Jason Poindexter III invited us to their home for dinner, which in itself was a thrill; but when we sat down to eat in their lovely formal dining room and were waited on by (do you call them servants?), I thought I was in another world.

I couldn't turn down any of those delectable offerings, could I? I've never hurt anyone's feelings, even mine, by turning down food. Should I start now?

As I surveyed the other guests, I noticed several ladies (the skinny ones) said,

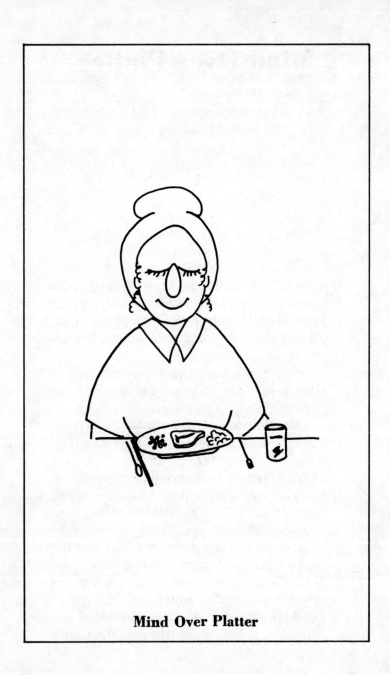

Mind Over Platter

"No, thank you," and they didn't even wince. I guessed I'd be able to refuse when it came my turn.

What an evening. The conversation was fascinating, the company delightful, the surroundings elegant, and the food was—well, the food was GREAT. And all praise to the Lord for helping me to be moderate.

I'm learning that it helps to decide, before eating out, just what and what not to put in that hole in my face. I had decided on vegetables, meat and salad. I passed on the bread, starches and, oh, it gives me great pain even now—the pastries. I didn't even look at them. And I left the dinner party feeling so good, yes, even a little proud.

So this is moderation, huh? Philippians 4:5 says, "Let your moderation be known unto all men." And I sure felt like shouting, "See, everybody? I'm moderate. Whooppee!" But then I remembered the rest of the verse, "The Lord is at hand." Just knowing He was there gave me encouragement and satisfaction. He knew I was moderate. He knew I wanted to please Him more than myself. That's what really matters.

Dear Friend

Maybe you've gotten into the habit of giving in to your wants, and it will be hard to learn moderation. But it can become a habit too. And just like any habit (good ones, that is) is hard to learn, it does get easier the more you practice it. And it makes you feel so good about yourself. It will be a testimony to others, too, of the power and presence of God as you "let your moderation be known unto all men," because, "the Lord is at hand."

Dear Lord

It's obvious that in the past
I've used no self-control
For I see around my waist
A great big fleshy roll!

More Food for Thought

"Whether therefore ye eat, or drink, or whatsoever ye do, do all to the glory of God" (I Corinthians 10:31).

". . . But if ye through the Spirit do mortify the deeds of the body, ye shall live" (Romans 8:13b).

Big Wheel

(Pride)

Dear Diary

It even hurts to smile today. But that isn't what hurts most. Yesterday I learned the truth of the words, "Pride goeth before a fall."

I'm afraid it went to my head when the kids said, "Mom, you've lost so much weight, you shouldn't be embarrassed about coming roller skating with us."

"Are you sure you want me to?" I asked, trying to hide the quiver in my voice.

"Yeah, it'll be lots of fun," they said, glancing sideways at each other.

"Well . . .," I stalled, "I haven't skated since high school days, but I was pretty good then." I took a deep breath, imagining myself as I was a few years ago (quite a few). "Okay, I'll go!"

The first half hour was traumatic; all that noise; all those kids; and those wheels on my feet. Oh, dear, what had I done?

But after letting my daughter pry me off the rail, my progress quickened.

Each time around the room of swirling figures, I felt more confidence. I caught a quick glimpse of myself in the huge mirror that covered one wall and was surprised to see how good I looked.

"Wow," I murmured, knowing I couldn't be heard over the din, "I'm okay —I really like the new, thinner ME. As I approached the mirror again, I decided to cross my feet like I saw the others doing, while watching my reflection.

CRASH! What happened? How did I get on the floor?

A little boy rushed over, but had to call several buddies to help drag me out of the pathway of the spinning, squealing boys and girls. (I guess I'm not the featherweight I thought I was.)

Oh-ow—everything hurt as I limped to the bench and gingerly sat . . . on my side. Oh, well, so I won't be the only middle-aged member of the Follies.

After thinking over the events of yesterday, I realize that I fell because I had my attention focused in the wrong place. You know, it's easy to become so pleased with your new image that pride can cause an even more serious fall.

"Look at me. See me walk. Watch me eat. I love me." When the attention is on self instead of Christ, look out. The Lord Jesus Christ is my life, and He should get

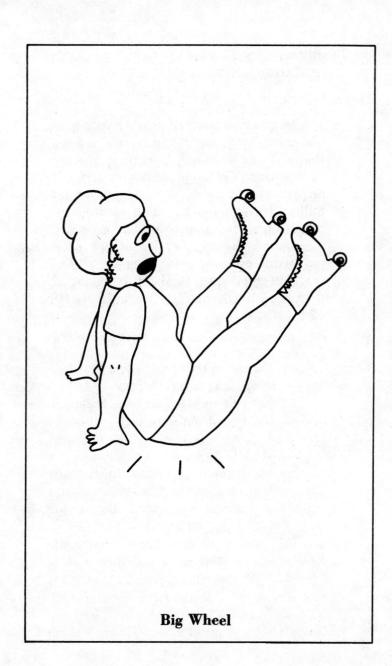

Big Wheel

all the glory.
Look at Him!

Dear Friend

As you find yourself nearing your goal, watch out for pride; it can erect a pedestal that will take you away from the fellowship of not only God, but also your friends. So ask God to give you the gift of humility, then you can live with yourself and others on a level that won't let you down.

Remember, humility is not just dropping your eyes—it's dropping your "I's."

"Let him that thinketh he standeth take heed lest he fall" (I Corinthians 10:12).

Dear Lord

I'm afraid that pride came in
And clouded up my eyes
For I thought I was doing great,
But I got a real surprise!

More Food for Thought

"For all that is in the world, the lust of the flesh, and the lust of the eyes, and the pride of life, is not of the Father, but is of the world" (I John 2:16).

"My soul shall make her boast in the LORD: the humble shall hear thereof, and be glad" (Psalm 34:2).

I Do

(Works)

Dear Diary

"There, there, don't cry, Betty. Here's a tissue for your nose." As she blew long and loud, I remembered that it was almost time to take my son to his trumpet lesson.

"But I know Jeff doesn't love me," she sniffed. "We've been married for a year, and he hardly ever tells me anymore." She blew again. "When I ask him if he loves me, he just grunts, 'Course, I do.' "

"See," I said, patting her hand, "he does love you."

"But I want to hear him say it."

"You know, Betty, I had a friend that gave the impression of having the perfect marriage. Her husband always held her hand or had his arm around her, giving her sweet little pecks on the cheek, no matter where they were.

"But when I heard they were having serious problems, she confided that all of his love was just 'show and tell.' He used their money on his own interests, and was mad when she bought something for herself. He didn't do anything around the house or yard, occupied himself in sports away from home, and never talked to her."

Betty's eyes brightened, "Well—Jeff does take good care of me. He tries to

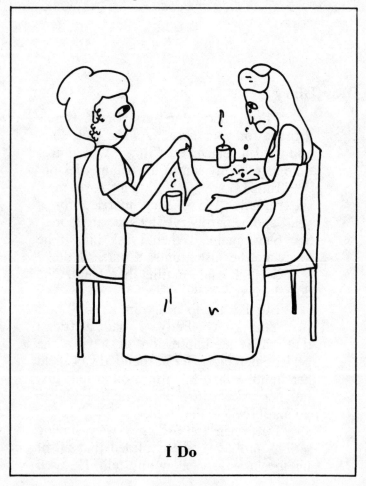

I Do

get anything I need. He's a great one to listen to my problems—and does all he can to make our home a warm and happy place."

"There, what did I tell you? Love is more than spewing—it's doing."

You know, it's not enough to say you will diet—you must *do-it*. I used to buy all the books on dieting and obesity I could find, hoping that if I read them faithfully, one day I would wake up thin. But it didn't work that way. I had to put my diet where my mouth was . . . so to speak.

Dear Friend

When you reach your goal, don't talk about how much you lost as you pile in the rich desserts. Be aware of what you're eating. Dieting is a lifetime deal; you can't relax and eat everything you want ever again—unless you want to be fat again. You'll have to use your self-control, for words are meaningful only when they're backed up with action.

Jesus reminded His followers that there were many who said, "Lord, Lord," but didn't do what He told them to. They were not His. He could tell the ones that really belonged to Him because they kept His commandments. Let's not fool ourselves into thinking we are His children because we belong to a church, or because we talk about God. We are His only if we have fulfilled His requirements.

1. "Believe on the Lord Jesus Christ, and thou shalt be saved" (Acts 16:31).

2. "As many as received him, to them gave he power to become the sons of God, even to them that believe on his name" (John 1:12).

3. "The wages of sin is death; but the gift of God is eternal life through Jesus Christ our Lord" (Romans 6:23).

Have you received that gift? Do you love Him? Then you will want to read His Word to find what you can do to please Him.

"But be ye doers of the word, and not hearers only, deceiving your own selves" (James 1:22).

Dear Lord

"Talk is cheap,"
I've heard it said.
My works must show
My faith's not dead.

More Food for Thought

"For by grace are ye saved through faith; and that not of yourselves: it is the gift of God: not of works, lest any man should boast. For we are his workmanship, created in Christ Jesus unto good works, which God hath before ordained that we should walk in them" (Ephesians 2:8-10).

Work, Work, Work

(Discipline)

Dear Diary

Housework isn't my favorite pastime, but every now and then (mostly then) I get a streak of ambition and accomplish more in one day than I usually do in a week—okay, a month. That's when I do the icky things like scooping out the winter's accumulation of ashes from the fireplace, cleaning the fan above the stove (ugh) and sweeping under the refrigerator. Yesterday's find was a Barbie doll shoe, two marbles, a popsicle stick, a soggy pretzel and about a pound of fuzz.

It's very easy for me to procrastinate when it comes to such unpleasant tasks, but I felt awfully proud when it was done, and took each member of the family by the hand to "show and tell." Strange, isn't it, when things are clean, no one notices; but when they're dirty . . .?

There are a few disagreeable jobs that need doing in my life too, like getting rid of some resentments, throwing out the desire to gossip, cleaning up on discouragement and self-pity and completely changing my eating habits; but I keep putting them off. I'm more aware of their presence than I was of the lint under the refrigerator, but I haven't the will to do something about it. How can I acquire the spiritual ambition to do some interior decorating? I need a push.

I know I can't just fold my hands and wait for a miracle; it doesn't happen that way. When I know something is amiss, I should go to the Bible and find God's directions.

Do I really want to be His disciple? Then I'm going to have to be *disciplined* and do what He says. I think I can use much the same equipment in cleaning up my character as I used in cleaning my house:

(1) the apron of discipline to cover my laziness,
(2) the water of the Word to wash away my sin,
(3) the broom of faith to sweep away doubts, and
(4) the dustcloth of obedience to wipe away self-will.

Someone has said, "Everything comes to him who waits, if he works while he waits."

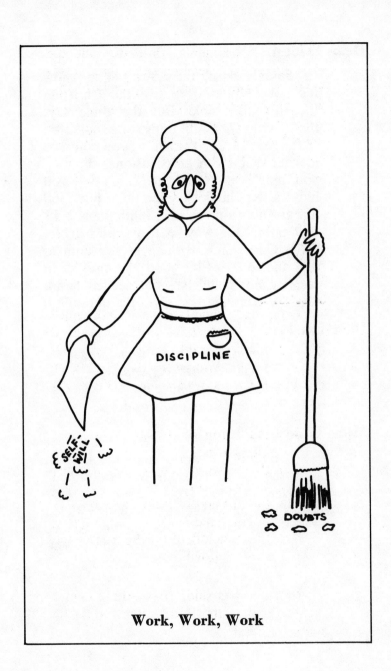

Work, Work, Work

Dear Friend

Sounds hard, doesn't it? You know it's not only hard to live the Christian life, it's impossible. But the Bible says that "with *God,* all things are possible" (Matthew 19:26b). Even as you continue in your diet (with an occasional slip-up), you may feel as defeated as when you have a big housecleaning job, but God has given us a promise in Philippians 2:13 that points the way to a disciplined life. "It is God which worketh in you both to *will* and to *do* of his good pleasure." You see, He not only gives the needed desire to serve Him, He also gives the durability.

Dear Lord

I'm asking You for something
I guess it's called gumption,
For if I don't have it
I simply can't function.

More Food for Thought

"Commit thy works unto the LORD, and thy thoughts shall be established" (Proverbs 16:3).

"Jesus answered and said unto them, This is the work of God, that ye believe on him whom he hath sent" (John 6:29).

A-One-And-A-Two-And-A-

(Exercise)

Dear Diary

"Teddy Bear, Teddy Bear, turn a. . . .
Teddy Bear, Teddy Bear, turn around.
Teddy Bear, Teddy. . . . Teddy Bear, Teddy Bear, turn around. Teddy Bear, Teddy
Bear, touch the gr. . . ."

I know that exercise is good for you,
but this is ridiculous. I used to jump rope
a lot when I was a kid, and I've seen my
children do it many times, but somehow,
I just can't get the gist of it anymore.

"Mom, I can't believe you," my daughter said, gently patting my arm, "you can't
jump to 'Teddy Bear' and turn the rope
yourself!"

"Oh, so that's where the trouble is,"
I answered, puffing out each word like a
corroded teakettle whistle.

She was right. It was much easier to
jump one-and-a-two-and-a-three-and-a-
four, and I didn't get so tangled up in the
rope.

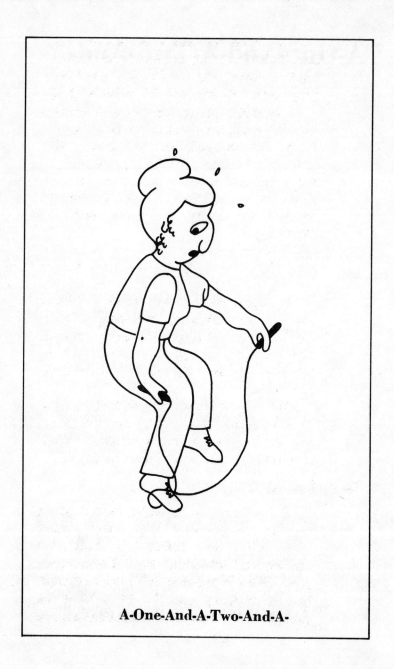

A-One-And-A-Two-And-A-

I've been jumping rope a little each day and increasing the length of time as I felt stronger; and you know, it's not only fun, I can feel my muscles tightening up.

I couldn't, or wouldn't have begun an exercise program those many pounds ago; I just felt too awkward and heavy. But since adhering to my diet long enough to see a big difference on the scale, as well as on the body, I feel so much better and stronger physically, I actually want to exercise.

Now let's see, how did that other one go? "Not-last-night-but-the-night-before . . ."

It seems to me that when a person eats a well-balanced, well-proportioned diet, the natural result is greater strength and therefore a will to get out and do something active. To put the machine in operation.

When I mentioned this to Les, he said, "You're right, honey, why don't you get out there and mow the front lawn?" Well, that isn't exactly what I had in mind.

Dear Friend

I imagine that as we've moved along together on our diets that you're feeling more active than before too. And have you noticed something else? These verses from God's Word that we've been committing to memory and the extra food for thought that helps us through the day, are making us stronger Christians.

The Bible is our spiritual food, and as we assimilate it into our lives, we become healthier spiritually. And not only that, don't you find you want to get out and share His Word with others? This is our spiritual exercise. Sharing our faith with those around us. It will keep us from becoming flabby followers, and will instead enable us to be dexterous disciples.

How about finding some form of exercise to begin today? Don't overdo it, though. Just a little at a time will strengthen you naturally.

And as far as this matter of witnessing or sharing God's Word with others is concerned, start with someone you know and like, and little by little your spiritual muscles will grow until you'll be sharing with all who hunger and thirst for a knowledge of Jesus Christ.

Dear Lord

> *Help me to hang in there*
> *If I make the wrong move*
> *While skipping the rope*
> *Or speaking of Your love.*

More Food for Thought

"And herein do I exercise myself, to have always a conscience void of offense toward God, and toward men" (Acts 24:16).

A Highway
Through the Desert

(Plateaus)

Dear Diary

"Whew, it's hot," I sputtered, pulling at the collar of my blouse and wiping my forehead. "Do you think we'll ever get out of this heat? We've been driving for hours and all I can see ahead is more desert." (Wish it were dessert, instead— nice mounds of ice cream in place of sand.)

"Sure, just be patient, honey. If we keep moving along this highway, we'll be in the mountains before you know it."

Ah, the mountains. I could imagine the fragrance of the pines and the cool, crisp air caressing my face. "Well, if you say so, but I sure don't see anything for miles but sand and sagebrush. Why don't we stop and rest awhile?"

"It'll just take that much longer to get there." Les smiled at me and added, "Why don't you put your head back and close your eyes. Just leave the driving to me, and we'll be out of here in no time."

He was right—my fretting and impatience were only an irritant to us both. As I began to relax to the hum of the motor and gentle vibrations of rubber on concrete, I remembered how impatient I had become with my diet about halfway through. I wasn't losing nearly as fast as I thought I should. I just stayed at the same weight, the scale moving down in tiny segments over a period of several weeks. How discouraging. I wanted to give up on the whole "schmier." All I could envision was a struggle of keeping "legal," with no results in view. But if I had given up, it would have taken me much longer to reach my destination than it has. Or I may never have reached it.

It was then someone told me about the plateaus in dieting. They said it was very important to continue on the same eating program and rest assured the goal would be reached. And it was true. Little by little the numbers began decreasing on the scale as well as on my dress labels.

Hmmm, what's that cool breeze blowing in the window?

"Hey, wake up, sleepyhead, we're out of the desert. Let's stop for something to eat—something on your diet, of course."

Dear Friend

If you haven't encountered this phenomenon yet, be prepared for it, so you

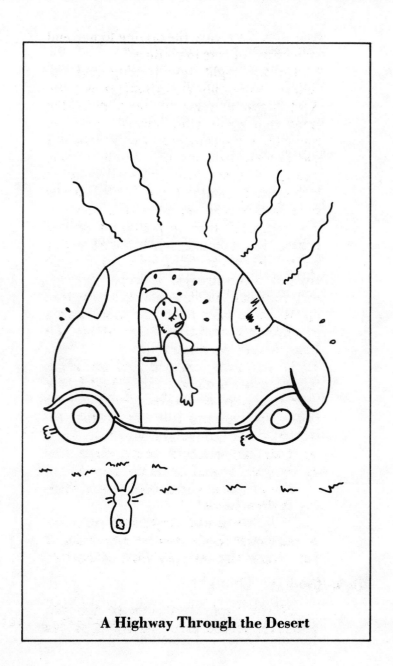

A Highway Through the Desert

won't become discouraged. Just keep on with the diet, as if you were traveling through the desert on a highway. It leads to your destination, and the closer you follow it, the sooner you'll be there.

Have you had any plateaus in your spiritual life? I have. There are times when nothing appears to be happening. God seems distant. In fact, you wonder if He hears your prayers at all. Problems don't get better, besetting sins are as strong, Bible study is dry and lifeless and there is no urge to tell others of the Living Christ. (How can there be when He doesn't seem to be living to us?)

Anyway, those plateaus or desert experiences are just a section we must travel through to reach the higher places. Don't give up your prayer and Bible study. Keep on. Rest in the Lord. Let Him take you through the dry times in your life. He travels the highway with us, leading to the high places in Christ Jesus.

What more could we ask?

Dear Lord

> *I need You to keep going*
> *When all around seems dreary*
> *For you know the Way*
> *And give strength to the weary.*

More Food for Thought

"Prepare ye the way of the LORD, make straight in the desert a highway for our God " (Isaiah 40:3).

From Here to Maternity

(Position)

Dear Diary

"What?" I gasped, feeling the blood rush from my face and come to rest somewhere near the pit of my stomach. "Say that again, Doctor. No, on second thought, don't say it again."

"Yes, Mrs. Cook, from my examination, there is no doubt—you will soon be welcoming another little 'Cookie' into your home."

Now don't get me wrong, it isn't that I don't love children. I do. Always have. In fact, you could say when God gave the commandment to Eve to "multiply and replenish the earth," I took it literally, and have added six, yes, 6 more adorable babies to our planet (my apologies to Planned Parenthood). But another one? After all, enough is enough.

My head began to reel as bright flashes of red and blue intertwined with my confused thoughts. "But I've almost reached my goal. I so wanted to be thin again. I've worked so hard at my diet. I already have children in college. Why?" The questions and whirling kaleidoscopic colors ended abruptly at the sound of loud music coming from somewhere above my head.

I opened my eyes as I automatically reached up to turn off the clock radio.

With an unrestrained, "Yippee!" I leaped out of bed, rubbing my tummy and pinching in my waist.

"What's the matter with you?" my husband grumbled from under his pillow. "It's not your birthday, is it?"

"No—but I sure feel like celebrating!"

One eye peered out of the covers, rolled up in disgust and closed again. I guess he didn't want to hear my dream.

Just a dream—but what if it were true, how would I have handled it? Many times in life when plans are changed, our whole life goes into a "tilt" position. Some problems are so serious that those confronted with them give up, consigned to defeat, living a meager day-to-day existence. Then there are those who simply can't take another setback, and decide to end it all. How sad.

Dear Friend

How is the Christian to face obstacles? Should we just muddle through, wearing a long face and mumbling, "It's just my cross to bear." Does a Christian have any

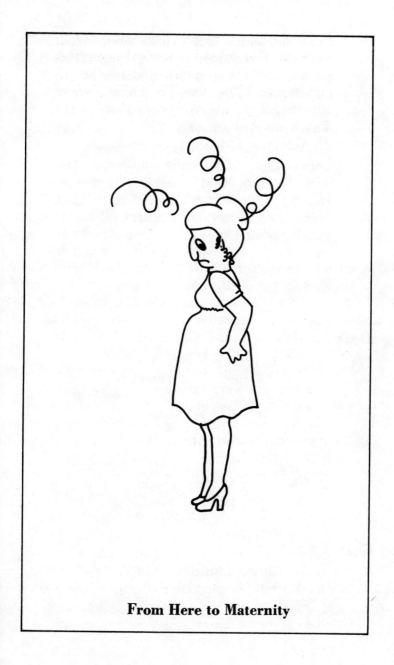

From Here to Maternity

right to respond to problems with, "Well, I guess I'm okay—under the circumstances." No, we are to live above the circumstances, "in the heavenlies where Christ sits at the right hand of God." That's our position, *in Him*.

We all have problems and changes that come unexpectedly and uninvited. But such "acts of God" shouldn't throw us; remember who we are—children of God, and where we are—in Christ. God knows exactly what is needed to help us mature to the place where we are conformed to the image of Christ, so dare we fight against His perfect plan for our lives?

Dear Lord

Help me to see beyond
The darkness of this day
And remember that you promised
To be with me alway.

More Food for Thought

"For I am persuaded, that neither death, nor life, nor angels, nor principalities, nor powers, nor things present, nor things to come, nor height, nor depth, nor any other creature, shall be able to separate us from the love of God, which is in Christ Jesus our Lord" (Romans 8:38,39).

Hidden Treasures

(Values)

Dear Diary

Danny, then only six years old, stood at the front door, a grin lighting his face. "Oh, Mom, you'll never guess what I've found. It's the bestest treasure I ever had!"

I looked down at my little "nature boy," perspiration running down his tanned face, and began to guess what "treasure" he had hidden behind his back.

"Let's see—a rock?"

"No."

"A flower?"

"No."

"Well, I think it must be something great to make you so happy. I give up. What is it?"

As he opened his little fists, I felt my hair stand on end, but managed a "Wow, I never would have guessed that!"

Filling up both hands and slithering through chubby fingers were CATER-

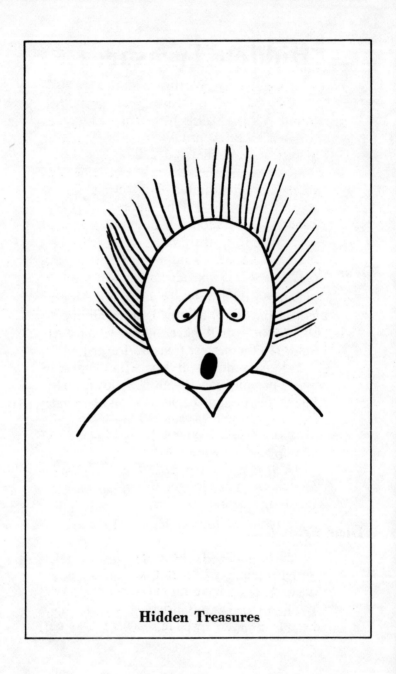

Hidden Treasures

PILLARS. Dozens of fat, hairy caterpillars.

"See, Mom. Worms with fur coats!"

Oh, they were treasures all right. We found a box, filled it with leaves and watched them eventually become beautiful Monarch butterflies.

At first glance, we may not recognize what is truly valuable. Take food, for instance (Thanks, I'd be glad to!). Most people would choose a hot fudge sundae over an apple. But which one really has more food value? And many feel it is only civilized to drink alcohol with a meal or to offer it when friends drop in. But water, fruit or vegetable juice would benefit their bodies rather than destroying their brain cells. So be a true friend.

And this diet is not so dull—a certain amount of bread, milk, fruit, vegetables and meat each day can only do me good. I'd be foolish to return to my former way of eating when I not only look better, but also feel better than I have in years.

Yes, even I have experienced a metamorphosis. I no longer feel like crawling, but flying!

Dear Friend

Our diets have been like hidden treasures to us, so let's not give them up—ever. And we have an even more precious treasure in Jesus Christ. When we first heard of Him, we may have thought,

"Well, if I become a Christian, I'll probably have to give up a lot. I'll have to go to church and deny myself everything I enjoy. Life will be empty."

But when we trusted Christ as our Saviour from sin, we found it was a whole new thing. As different as a butterfly from a caterpillar. Life became full and rich. Eternity became real. Heaven became our new home. Circumstances and troubles became meaningful. Strangers became brothers and sisters, and best of all, God became our Father. Oh, what a treasure we who know Jesus Christ possess. Let's not only prize it above all other riches, but share it with those who are still crawling.

Dear Lord

> *I no longer cling to earth*
> *As a lowly (and fat) worm*
> *But fly through each day*
> *With faith steadfast and firm.*

More Food for Thought

"But lay up for yourselves treasures in heaven, where neither moth nor rust doth corrupt, and where thieves do not break through nor steal: For where your treasure is, there will your heart be also" (Matthew 6:20,21).

Love Story

(Love)

Dear Diary

"Mom, I'll do anything you say from now on," nine-year-old Barby announced, throwing her arms around my neck.

"What do you mean, honey?"

"Well, when you tell me to go to bed, I'll do it without arguing; and if you ask me to take out the garbage, I'll do it right away. I just love you so!"

Wow. In all my years of mothering, this was the best offer I'd ever had. Let's see. I could have her scrub the floors, pull weeds, clean out the cat-box. No, I wouldn't think up unpleasant tasks for her to do. I'd treat her offer fairly and be very careful of my requirements.

"Oh, Mom," she called over her shoulder as she breezed out the door, "is it okay if I start next week?"

How like me in my dedication to the Lord. I tell Him that I love Him, and I do; but I continually put off or drag my feet doing the things I know will please Him. In fact, sometimes when I get around to obeying the Lord, I do it with the feeling that I'm making a sacrifice.

I love the story in the Old Testament of King David and the time he looked down on his home town of Bethlehem, and longed for a drink of water from the well. He had been through many battles and troubles, and that water from Bethlehem would not only soothe his parched throat, but also his tired, parched spirit. Three of his soldiers risked their lives to go into enemy territory to bring back the cup of water to their king. David looked at it, looked at the men who had shown such love for him, and knew it was too precious to drink. Then he made an offering to the Lord (he didn't consider it a sacrifice), and poured the water out on the ground as an act of love for his God. There was no spirit of the martyr in David's action, only love. You can read it for yourself in II Samuel 23:14-17.

As I prayed this morning, asking God to help me to stay on my diet, I suddenly realized that I thought it was a great sacrifice for me to give up some of my natural desires for food. I have played the martyr many times when I turned down a second helping, or a piece of pie, instead of finding pleasure in obeying my Lord. I know that if I think I'm sacrificing or obeying

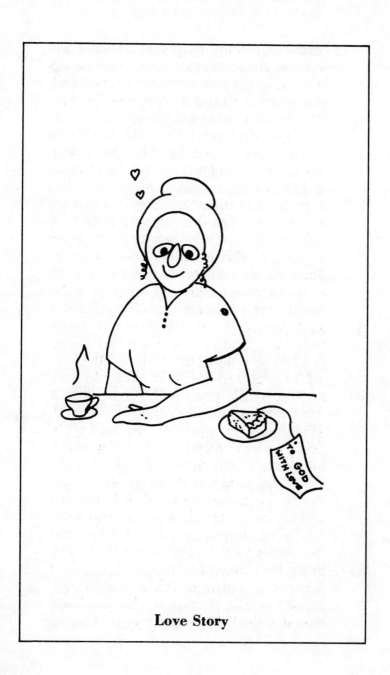

Love Story

God out of duty rather than love, I will very likely rebel when I've reached my goal, and begin eating anything and everything again. And get fat—again.

The motive for my being thin has to be right (if I want it to last, and have eternal benefits). It can't be that I want to be pretty—that would take more than a diet. Or that I want better health—I can lose that at any time. Or even to make my husband proud of me—he already is. My motive must be as pure as Barby's (but without hidden clauses), that I love my Father and want to please Him. And He will not abuse my love, but will gently and lovingly lead me in His way.

Dear Friend

Let's do as David, the man after God's own heart, did and give up those delicacies that mean so much to us, for the love of God. Make it a spiritual offering as you deny it to your own body. He will see your motive and be pleased.

Dear Lord

From this day on
I want to obey
Because I love You
And choose Your way.

More Food for Thought

". . . For the Lord seeth not as man seeth; for man looketh on the outward appearance, but the Lord looketh on the heart" (I Samuel 16:7).

Out of the Mouths
of Babes

(Simplicity)

Dear Diary

"Teacher, when you smile, your face gets all wrinkly."

"Do you have a plastic tooth?"

"Boy, teacher, you look like you need braces."

"My mother said it was about time you went on a diet!"

Just a few "adorable?" things said by my young Sunday School students. They certainly have a way of keeping a person humble, don't they?

But that's one of the things I like about kids, even though sometimes it smarts a bit. They see us as we are, not as we'd like to be seen. Their simplicity and honesty is something to protect and nurture; it's lost too soon anyway. In only a few short years, they'll have learned deceit and when to candy-coat their thoughts in order to assuage adults.

But it's that very simplicity and childlikeness the Lord Jesus commended when He said, "Whosoever shall not receive the kingdom of God as a little child shall in no wise enter therein" (Luke 18:17). How readily these young ones accept the truths of the gospel. Their openness to the love of Jesus Christ is, as yet, untouched by the cynicism of the world, and they respond happily and willingly to His invitation., "Suffer the little children to come unto me, and forbid them not: for of such is the kingdom of God" (Mark 10:14).

I want to be more like a child in my trust of the Saviour. My life should no longer be centered around such concerns as, "What shall I eat (that's rich and satisfying) or what shall I wear (that will make me look thinner) or where will I go tomorrow (an all-you-can-eat place?); but I should have an unaffected and uncluttered trust in the One who controls not only my tomorrows, but also my todays. This kind of simplicity will leave one free to enjoy life to the fullest, yet, tempered with Christ's wisdom, aware of the pitfalls and temptations.

Dear Friend

We've come a long way together on our diets and in our Christian walk since beginning this diary. I hope you feel the oneness with me that I feel with you. As children of God, we need each other for encouragement and enlightenment along

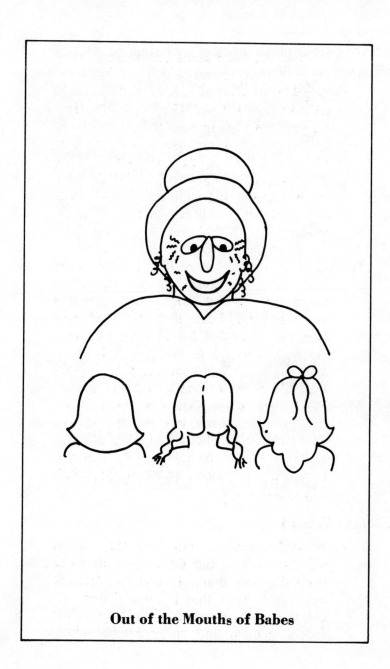

Out of the Mouths of Babes

our paths, whether we have a weight problem or not. There are many burdens being borne by those around us, and it's our privilege to help carry the load, making someone's pilgrimage here a more pleasant one.

Let's live Christ simply and honestly as children, yet bear our burdens with the strength and endurance of mature adults. ". . . but now are ye light in the Lord: walk as children of light" (Ephesians 5:8).

Dear Lord

Gentle Jesus, meek and mild,
Look upon this little child.
Pity my simplicity,
Suffer me to come to Thee.

(This was the child's prayer my mother taught me.)

More Food for Thought

"Little children, keep yourselves from idols" (I John 5:21).

"Ye are all the children of God by faith in Christ Jesus" (Galatians 3:26).

Watch Your Beginnings

(The End?)

Dear Diary

I stepped on the scale. Could it be true? I stepped off—then on—off—then an again. I had to be sure. "I'm not dreaming, am I?" I asked my reflection in the full-length mirror. It's true. I flung the door open and whooped, "I made it. I reached my goal. I'm thin!"

The whole family crowded into the tiny bathroom and looked at the numbers recorded on the scale.

"Right on, Mom."

"Fantastic."

"Great."

"Really."

"Neat."

"Oh, my thin Mommy."

"You're beautiful, sweetheart," my husband said as he picked me up (yes, ME), and carried me into the living room amidst squealing and laughing. Then he sat down, me on his lap. As the children dispersed to gobble down breakfasts, gather up books and gawk around the corner, Les gave me some "words of advice."

"Now, honey, you've proven not only to us, but more importantly to yourself, that you could eat yourself thin. Now think of this accomplishment, not as an end to your diet, but as a beginning of a new way of life."

A beginning. Hmm, I like it. It sounds fresh and new. And if I think of it as THE END, I may get right back into my old eating habits; but as a beginning, I can go on practicing self-control, still depending on the Lord's strength, and growing, not physically but spiritually, and emotionally, into the person God wants me to be.

Our pastor has said many times, "Watch your beginnings." By that he means, if you start off wrong whether it's a new day or a new endeavor, the end result will be wrong.

Dear Friend

Let's determine to "watch our beginnings." As each new day arrives, meet it with the Lord. Commit your appetite as well as your involvements to Him. If you haven't reached your goal yet—don't stop now. Go back and read these diary entries over again, allowing God's Word to strengthen and keep you till you reach your "beginning."

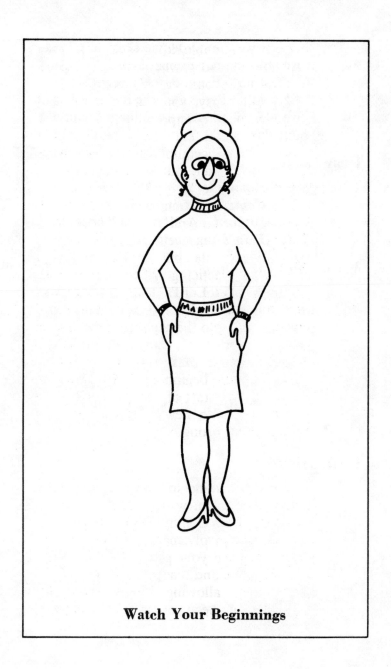

Watch Your Beginnings

"For we are made partakers of Christ, if we hold the beginning of our confidence steadfast unto the end" (Hebrews 3:14).

Now that I've gotten the body in shape, I wonder if there's something I can do about this nose?

Dear Lord

A new day so fresh and clean
Comes as a gift from Thee.
So Lord, I quickly give it back
That Thou canst keep for me.

More Food for Thought

"It is of the LORD'S mercies that we are not consumed, because His compassions fail not. They are new every morning: great is thy faithfulness" (Lamentations 3:22,23).

THE BEGINNING